ACID REFLUX RECIPE COOKBOOK

ANN DAVIS

TABLE OF CONTENTS

A persistent illness known as GERD causes stomach contents, such as acid, to reflux up into the esophagus. If treatment is not received, symptoms may worsen and cause damage to the esophagus. GERD is characterized by recurrent, chronic symptoms that happen at least twice a week. Even while heartburn and acid reflux are common names for GERD, they actually indicate quite distinct things.

SYMPTOMS OF GERD OR HEARTBURN

Heartburn is a burning feeling in the chest that normally gets worse when you're sleeping or right after eating.

- Acidic or sour taste in the mouth
- Coughing
- Vocal cord inflammation (laryngitis)
- Difficulty swallowing

- A lump in the throat sensation

FOOD TO CONSUME.

If you experience GERD (Gastroesophageal Reflux Disease), you should focus on consuming foods that are less likely to trigger acid reflux symptoms. Here's a list of foods that are generally considered safe to eat with GERD:

1. Non-acidic fruits: Bananas, apples, melons, pears, berries (except citrus fruits like oranges and lemons).
2. Vegetables: Broccoli, carrots, green beans, peas, spinach, kale, cauliflower (avoid tomatoes and onions).
3. Lean proteins: Skinless poultry, fish (like salmon and trout), tofu, lean cuts of beef or pork (avoid fried or fatty meats).

4. Whole grains: Oats, brown rice, quinoa, whole wheat bread, whole grain pasta (avoid refined grains and white bread).

5. Dairy: Low-fat or fat-free milk, yogurt, cheese (avoid full-fat dairy products).

6. Healthy fats: Olive oil, avocado, nuts, seeds (in moderation).

7. Herbs and spices: Ginger, turmeric, parsley, basil, cilantro (avoid spicy or peppery seasonings).

8. Beverages: Water, herbal teas (like chamomile or ginger tea), almond milk (avoid caffeinated beverages, carbonated drinks, and citrus juices).

9. Low-acid foods: Egg whites, oatmeal, non-citrus fruit juices (like apple or pear juice).

10. Healthy snacks: Rice cakes, pretzels, low-fat popcorn, vegetable sticks with hummus.

It is crucial for a patient to consider eating habits and portion sizes. Symptoms of GERD can be controlled by eating smaller meals throughout the day, avoid eating before going to bed and practicing mindful eating. Additionally, keep a food diary to track which foods trigger symptoms can be helpful in identifying and avoiding potential triggers. Always consult with a medical doctor or health care professional or a registered dietitian for personalized dietary advice and management of GERD.

PASTA RECIPES

1. Zucchini Noodles with Turkey Meatballs

Ingredients:

- 2 medium zucchinis
- 1 pound ground turkey
- 1/4 cup breadcrumbs (preferably whole grain)
- 1/4 cup grated Parmesan cheese
- 1 egg
- 2 cloves garlic, minced
- 1 teaspoon dried oregano
- Salt and pepper to taste
- 2 cups marinara sauce (low-acid or homemade)
- 1 tablespoon olive oil

Instructions:

1. Preheat the oven to 375°F (190°C).

2. Start by making the turkey meatballs. In a large bowl, combine ground turkey, breadcrumbs, Parmesan cheese, egg, minced garlic, dried oregano, salt, and pepper. Stir thoroughly to ensure that all ingredients are combined very well.

3. Shape the ingredients into meatballs with a diameter of about one inch each.

4. In a big pot or skillet, heat the oil on medium to relatively low heat. After it is hot, add the meatballs and simmer for about five minutes, or until it is brown all over.

5. Transfer the browned meatballs to a baking dish and pour marinara sauce over them.

6. Bake the meatballs for 20 to 25 minutes, or until they are well cooked, do this in a preheated oven.

7. While the meatballs are baking, prepare the zucchini noodles. Using a spiralizer or a

vegetable peeler, create noodles from the zucchinis.

8. In a big pan or skillet, heat the oil on medium to relatively low heat. Add the zucchini noodles and sauté for 2-3 minutes until tender but still slightly firm.

9. Once the meatballs are done baking, serve them over the zucchini noodles and garnish with additional Parmesan cheese if desired.

2. Salmon and Spinach Pasta

Ingredients:

- 8 ounces whole grain pasta (such as penne or spaghetti)
- 2 tablespoons olive oil
- 2 cloves garlic, minced

- 1 pound fresh salmon fillet, skin removed and cut into chunks
- Salt and pepper to taste
- 4 cups fresh spinach leaves
- 1/4 cup low-fat Greek yogurt
- 1 tablespoon lemon juice
- 1/4 cup grated Parmesan cheese

Instructions:

1. Follow the directions on the packaged to cook the whole grain pasta. Drain and set aside.
2. In a big pan or skillet, heat the oil on medium to relatively low heat. Add minced garlic and cook for 1 minute until fragrant.
3. Season the salmon chunks with salt and pepper, then add them to the skillet. Cook

for 4-5 minutes, stirring occasionally, until the salmon is cooked through.

4. Add fresh spinach leaves to the skillet and cook until wilted, about 2 minutes.

5. Reduce the heat to low and stir in Greek yogurt and lemon juice until well combined.

6. Add the cooked pasta to the skillet and toss everything together until evenly coated.

7. Cook for an additional 2-3 minutes until heated through.

8. Remove from heat and sprinkle grated Parmesan cheese over the pasta before serving.

3. Shrimp and Asparagus Pasta

Ingredients:

- 8 ounces whole wheat spaghetti

- 1 pound shrimp, peeled and deveined
- One bunch of asparagus, shredded
- 2 tablespoons olive oil
- 3 cloves garlic, minced
- 1/4 teaspoon red pepper flakes (optional)
- Salt and pepper to taste
- 1/4 cup low-sodium chicken broth
- 1 tablespoon lemon juice
- 1/4 cup grated Parmesan cheese

Instructions:

1. Cook the whole wheat spaghetti according to the package instructions. Drain and set aside.
2. In a big pan or skillet, heat the oil on medium to relatively low heat. Add minced garlic and red pepper flakes (if using) and cook for 1 minute.

3. Add shrimp to the skillet and cook until pink and opaque, about 3-4 minutes.

4. Add asparagus to the skillet and season with salt and pepper. Cook for an additional 3-4 minutes until asparagus is tender-crisp.

5. Pour in chicken broth and lemon juice, stirring to combine. Cook for another 1-2 minutes.

6. Add the cooked spaghetti to the skillet and toss everything together until well coated.

7. To serve, top the pasta with grated parmesan cheese.

4. Chicken Alfredo Pasta with Broccoli

Ingredients:

- 8 ounces whole grain fettuccine
- 2 boneless, skinless chicken breasts, diced

- 2 tablespoons olive oil
- 2 cloves garlic, minced
- 1 cup broccoli florets
- 1 cup low-fat milk
- 2 tablespoons whole wheat flour
- 1/4 cup grated Parmesan cheese
- Salt and pepper to taste

Instructions:

1. Cook the whole grain fettuccine according to the package instructions. Drain and set aside.
2. In a big pan or skillet, heat the oil on medium to relatively low heat. After adding the minced garlic, sauté for one minute.
3. Add diced chicken to the skillet and cook until browned and cooked through, about 5-6 minutes.

4. Add broccoli florets to the skillet and cook until tender, about 3-4 minutes.

5. In a small bowl, whisk together low-fat milk and whole wheat flour until smooth.

6. Pour the milk mixture into the skillet, stirring constantly, until the sauce thickens, about 2-3 minutes.

7. Stir in grated Parmesan cheese until melted and smooth.

8. Add the cooked fettuccine to the skillet and toss everything together until well coated. Adjust seasoning with salt and pepper if needed before serving.

5. Veggie Pesto Pasta

Ingredients:

- 8 ounces whole wheat spaghetti

- 1 cup cherry tomatoes, halved
- 1 cup baby spinach leaves
- 1/2 cup sliced black olives
- 1/4 cup pine nuts, toasted
- 1/4 cup grated Parmesan cheese
- Salt and pepper to taste
- 1/4 cup prepared pesto sauce

Instructions:

1. Cook the whole wheat spaghetti according to the package instructions. Drain and set aside.
2. In a large mixing bowl, combine cooked spaghetti, cherry tomatoes, baby spinach leaves, sliced black olives, and toasted pine nuts.

3. Add grated Parmesan cheese, salt, and pepper to the bowl and toss everything together.

4. Drizzle prepared pesto sauce over the pasta and toss again until well coated.

5. Serve immediately, garnished with additional Parmesan cheese if desired.

6. Turkey and Vegetable Stir-Fry Noodles

Ingredients:

- 8 ounces whole wheat spaghetti
- 1 tablespoon sesame oil
- 1 pound ground turkey
- 1 onion, sliced
- 1 bell pepper, sliced
- 1 zucchini, sliced
- 2 cups broccoli florets

- 3 cloves garlic, minced
- 1/4 cup low-sodium soy sauce
- 2 tablespoons rice vinegar
- 1 tablespoon honey
- 1 teaspoon grated ginger
- 2 green onions, chopped (for garnish)

Instructions:

1. Cook the whole wheat spaghetti according to the package instructions. Drain and set aside.
2. In a big pan or skillet, heat the sesame oil on medium to relatively low heat. Add ground turkey and cook until browned, breaking it up with a spatula, about 5-6 minutes.
3. Add sliced onion, bell pepper, zucchini, and broccoli florets to the skillet. Cook, stirring

frequently, until vegetables are tender-crisp, about 4-5 minutes.

4. Add minced garlic to the skillet and cook for 1 minute until fragrant.

5. In a small bowl, whisk together low-sodium soy sauce, rice vinegar, honey, and grated ginger.

6. Cover the veggies and turkey in the skillet with the sauce. Stir to ensure even coating.

7. Add the cooked spaghetti to the skillet and toss everything together until well combined.

8. Cook for an additional 2-3 minutes until heated through.

9. Garnish with chopped green onions before serving.

7. Caprese Pasta Salad

Ingredients:

- 8 ounces whole wheat rotini pasta
- 1 cup cherry tomatoes, halved
- 1 cup fresh mozzarella balls (ciliegine), halved
- 1/4 cup chopped fresh basil leaves
- 2 tablespoons balsamic glaze
- 2 tablespoons olive oil
- Salt and pepper to taste

Instructions:

1. Cook the whole wheat rotini pasta according to the package instructions. Drain and rinse under cold water.
2. In a large mixing bowl, combine cooked pasta, cherry tomatoes, fresh mozzarella balls, and chopped fresh basil leaves.

3. Drizzle balsamic glaze and olive oil over the pasta salad. Add salt and pepper according to the taste you want.
4. Toss everything together until well combined.
5. Serve chilled or at room temperature.

8. Lentil and Vegetable Pasta

Ingredients:

- 8 ounces whole grain spaghetti
- 1 cup cooked lentils
- 1 cup diced carrots
- 1 cup diced zucchini
- 1 cup diced bell peppers (any color)
- 1/2 cup diced onion
- 2 cloves garlic, minced
- 2 tablespoons olive oil

- 1 teaspoon Italian seasoning
- Salt and pepper to taste
- 1/4 cup grated Parmesan cheese

Instructions:

1. Cook the whole grain spaghetti according to the package instructions. Drain and set aside.
2. In a big pan or skillet, heat the oil on medium to relatively low heat. Add diced onion and cook until translucent, about 3-4 minutes.
3. Add minced garlic to the skillet and cook for 1 minute until fragrant.
4. Add diced carrots, zucchini, and bell peppers to the skillet. Cook, stirring occasionally, until vegetables are tender, about 5-6 minutes.

5. Stir in cooked lentils and Italian seasoning. Cook for an additional 2-3 minutes to heat through.

6. Add the cooked spaghetti to the skillet and toss everything together until well combined.

7. Season with salt and pepper to taste.

8. Serve hot, garnished with grated Parmesan cheese.

9. Spinach and Ricotta Stuffed Shells

Ingredients:

- 8 ounces jumbo pasta shells
- 2 cups fresh spinach leaves, chopped
- 1 cup low-fat ricotta cheese
- 1/4 cup grated Parmesan cheese
- 1 egg

- 2 cloves garlic, minced
- 1/4 teaspoon nutmeg
- Salt and pepper to taste
- 2 cups marinara sauce (low-acid or homemade)

Instructions:

1. Follow the directions on the package to cook the pasta shells. Drain and set aside.
2. Preheat the oven to 375°F (190°C).
3. In a mixing bowl, combine chopped fresh spinach, low-fat ricotta cheese, grated Parmesan cheese, egg, minced garlic, nutmeg, salt, and pepper. Stir thoroughly to ensure that all ingredients are combined equally.
4. Stuff each cooked pasta shell with the spinach and ricotta mixture.

5. Line the bottom of a baking dish with a thin layer of marinara sauce.

6. Arrange the stuffed shells in the baking dish in a single layer.

7. Once the stuffed shells are evenly covered, pour the leftover marinara sauce over them.

8. Cover the baking dish with foil and bake in the preheated oven for 25-30 minutes, or until the shells are heated through and the sauce is bubbly.

9. Take out of the oven and allow it to cool down a little before serving.

10. Tuna and White Bean Pasta Salad

Ingredients:

- 8 ounces whole wheat fusilli pasta
- 1 can of white beans, washed and sieved

- 1 can of tuna in water, sieved
- 1 cup cherry tomatoes, halved
- 1/4 cup chopped fresh parsley
- 2 tablespoons olive oil
- 2 tablespoons lemon juice
- 1 teaspoon Dijon mustard
- Salt and pepper to taste

Instructions:

1. Cook the whole wheat fusilli pasta according to the package instructions. Drain and rinse under cold water.
2. In a large mixing bowl, combine cooked pasta, white beans, tuna, cherry tomatoes, and chopped fresh parsley.
3. In a small bowl, whisk together olive oil, lemon juice, Dijon mustard, salt, and pepper to make the dressing.

4. Pour the dressing over the pasta salad and toss everything together until well coated.

5. Serve chilled or at room temperature.

BREAKFAST

1. Oatmeal with Bananas and Almond Butter

Ingredients:

- 1/2 cup rolled oats
- 1 cup water or non-dairy milk
- 1 ripe banana, sliced
- 1 tablespoon almond butter
- 1 tablespoon honey (optional)
- Pinch of cinnamon

Instructions:

1. In a small saucepan, bring water or non-dairy milk to a boil.

2. Stir in rolled oats and reduce heat to a simmer. Stir continuously until the oats become creamy about 5 to 7 minutes.

3. Switch off the source of the heat and pour the oatmeal in a bowl.

4. Top with sliced bananas, almond butter, a drizzle of honey (if desired), and a pinch of cinnamon.

5. Serve warm and enjoy!

2. Greek Yogurt Parfait

Ingredients:

- 1/2 cup plain Greek yogurt
- 1/4 cup granola (low-acid or homemade)
- 1/4 cup mixed berries (such as strawberries, blueberries, or raspberries)
- 1 tablespoon honey (optional)

Instructions:

1. In a glass or bowl, layer plain Greek yogurt, granola, and mixed berries.
2. Drizzle with honey if desired.
3. Repeat layering if making multiple servings.
4. Serve immediately and enjoy this refreshing and nutritious parfait.

3. Scrambled Tofu Breakfast Bowl

Ingredients:

- 1/2 block firm tofu, crumbled
- 1/4 cup diced bell peppers
- 1/4 cup diced tomatoes
- 1/4 cup diced mushrooms
- 1/4 teaspoon turmeric
- Salt and pepper to taste

- 1 tablespoon olive oil
- Chopped fresh parsley for garnish

Instructions:

1. In a big pan or skillet, heat the oil on medium to relatively low heat. Add diced bell peppers, tomatoes, and mushrooms to the skillet. Sauté until vegetables are tender.
2. Add crumbled tofu to the skillet and sprinkle with turmeric, salt, and pepper. Cook for 3-5 minutes, stirring occasionally, until tofu is heated through and slightly golden.
3. Remove from heat and transfer scrambled tofu and vegetables to a bowl.
4. Garnish with chopped fresh parsley and serve warm.

4. Whole Grain Toast with Avocado and Tomato

Ingredients:

- 2 slices whole grain bread, toasted
- 1/2 ripe avocado, mashed
- 1 small tomato, sliced
- Salt and pepper to taste
- Optional toppings: red pepper flakes, chopped fresh herbs

Instructions:

1. Toast whole grain bread until golden brown.
2. Spread mashed avocado evenly on each slice of toast.
3. Add sliced tomatoes on top and season with salt and pepper.
4. Add optional toppings such as red pepper flakes or chopped fresh herbs if desired.

5. Serve immediately and enjoy this simple yet satisfying breakfast.

5. Smoothie Bowl

Ingredients:

- 1 ripe banana, frozen
- 1/2 cup frozen mixed berries
- 1/2 cup spinach leaves
- 1/2 cup plain Greek yogurt
- 1/4 cup almond milk (or any non-citrus non-dairy milk)
- Toppings to add: granola, sliced banana, shredded coconut, chia seeds

Instructions:

1. In a blender, combine frozen banana, frozen mixed berries, spinach leaves, plain Greek yogurt, and almond milk.

2. To get the right consistency, add extra almond milk if necessary and blend until smooth and creamy.

3. Pour the smoothie into a bowl.

4. Top with granola, sliced banana, shredded coconut, and chia seeds.

5. Serve immediately and enjoy this nutritious and refreshing breakfast option.

6. Veggie Breakfast Burrito

Ingredients:

- 2 large eggs
- 1/4 cup diced bell peppers
- 1/4 cup diced onions

- 1/4 cup diced tomatoes
- 2 tablespoons shredded cheese (optional)
- 1 whole grain tortilla
- 1 tablespoon olive oil
- Salt and pepper to taste
- Salsa or avocado for serving (optional)

Instructions:

1. In a big pan or skillet, heat the oil on medium to relatively low heat.
2. Add diced bell peppers, onions, and tomatoes to the skillet. Sauté until vegetables are tender.
3. In a separate bowl, whisk eggs with salt and pepper.
4. Pour beaten eggs into the skillet with the sautéed vegetables. Cook, stirring occasionally, until eggs are scrambled and cooked through.

5. Sprinkle shredded cheese (if using) over the scrambled eggs and let it melt.

6. Warm the whole grain tortilla in a separate skillet or microwave.

7. Put the veggie mixture and scrambled eggs in to the tortilla.

8. Fold up the tortilla to create a burrito.

9. If you prefer, top with avocado slices or salsa.

7. Blueberry Chia Seed Pudding

Ingredients:

- 1/4 cup chia seeds
- 1 cup almond milk (or any non-citrus non-dairy milk)
- 1/2 teaspoon vanilla extract
- 1 tablespoon maple syrup (optional)

- 1/4 cup fresh blueberries

Instructions:

1. In a mixing bowl, whisk together chia seeds, almond milk, vanilla extract, and maple syrup (if using).
2. Let the mixture sit for 5 minutes, then whisk again to break up any clumps of chia seeds.
3. Cover the bowl and refrigerate for at least 2 hours or overnight, allowing the chia seeds to absorb the liquid and thicken into a pudding-like consistency.
4. Once the chia seed pudding has set, stir in fresh blueberries.
5. Serve chilled and enjoy this nutritious and fiber-rich breakfast option.

8. Sweet Potato Hash

Ingredients:

- 1 medium sweet potato, peeled and diced
- 1/2 cup diced bell peppers
- 1/4 cup diced onions
- 2 cloves garlic, minced
- 1 tablespoon olive oil
- Salt and pepper to taste
- Optional toppings: sliced avocado, poached eggs

Instructions:

1. In a big pan or skillet, heat the oil on medium to relatively low heat.
2. Add diced sweet potatoes to the skillet and cook, stirring occasionally, until golden brown and tender.

3. Add diced bell peppers, onions, and minced garlic to the skillet. Sauté until vegetables are tender.

4. Season with salt and pepper.

5. Serve sweet potato hash on its own or topped with sliced avocado or poached eggs for added protein.

9. Cottage Cheese Pancakes

Ingredients:

- 1/2 cup cottage cheese
- 2 large eggs
- 1/4 cup whole wheat flour
- 1/4 teaspoon baking powder
- 1/2 teaspoon vanilla extract
- Pinch of salt

- Olive oil or non-stick cooking spray for cooking

Instructions:

1. In a blender, combine cottage cheese, eggs, whole wheat flour, baking powder, vanilla extract, and a pinch of salt. Blend until smooth.
2. Heat olive oil or non-stick cooking spray in a skillet over medium heat.
3. Pour batter onto the skillet to form pancakes.
4. Cook until bubbles form on the surface of the pancakes, then flip and cook until golden brown on the other side.
5. Serve pancakes warm with your choice of toppings such as fresh fruit, honey, or Greek yogurt.

10. Breakfast Quinoa Bowl

Ingredients:

- 1/2 cup cooked quinoa
- 1/2 cup mixed berries
- 1 tablespoon almond butter
- 1 tablespoon of honey (optional)
- 1 tablespoon of chopped nuts
- Pinch of cinnamon

Instructions:

1. In a bowl, combine cooked quinoa with mixed berries.
2. Drizzle almond butter and honey (if using) over the quinoa and berries.
3. Sprinkle with chopped nuts and a pinch of cinnamon.

4. This breakfast bowl is full of protein and is
    best served warm.

DINNER

1. Baked Salmon with Lemon and Herbs

Ingredients:

- 4 salmon fillets
- 2 tablespoons olive oil
- 2 cloves garlic, minced
- 1 tablespoon chopped fresh dill
- 1 tablespoon chopped fresh parsley
- 1 lemon, thinly sliced
- Salt and pepper to taste

Instructions:

1. Preheat the oven to 375°F (190°C).
2. Arrange the salmon fillets on a parchment paper-lined baking pan.

3. Drizzle olive oil over the salmon and sprinkle with minced garlic, chopped dill, and chopped parsley.

4. Place slices of lemon over the fish.

5. Season with salt and pepper to taste.

6. Bake in the preheated oven for 12-15 minutes, or until salmon is cooked through and flakes easily with a fork.

7. Serve hot with a side of salad or streaming veggies.

2. Grilled Chicken Breast with Roasted Vegetables

Ingredients:

- 4 boneless, skinless chicken breasts
- 2 tablespoons olive oil
- 2 cloves garlic, minced
- 1 teaspoon dried thyme

- 1 teaspoon dried rosemary
- 1 teaspoon dried oregano
- Salt and pepper to taste
- Assorted vegetables (such as bell peppers, zucchini, and cherry tomatoes), chopped

Instructions:

1. Preheat the grill to medium-high heat.
2. In a small bowl, mix together olive oil, minced garlic, dried thyme, dried rosemary, and dried oregano.
3. Brush the chicken breasts with the herb mixture and season with salt and pepper.
4. Place chicken breasts on the grill and cook for 6-8 minutes per side, or until cooked through.
5. Meanwhile, toss chopped vegetables with olive oil, salt, and pepper.

6. Place vegetables on a baking sheet and roast in the oven at 400°F (200°C) for 20-25 minutes, or until tender.

7. Serve grilled chicken breasts with roasted vegetables on the side.

3. Vegetable Stir-Fry with Tofu

Ingredients:

- 14 ounces firm tofu, drained and cubed
- 2 tablespoons soy sauce (low-sodium)
- 1 tablespoon sesame oil
- 2 tablespoons olive oil
- 2 cloves garlic, minced
- 1 teaspoon grated ginger
- Assorted vegetables (such as bell peppers, broccoli, and snap peas), chopped
- Cooked brown rice or quinoa for serving

Instructions:

1. In a small bowl, marinate tofu cubes in soy sauce and sesame oil for 15-20 minutes.
2. In a big pan or skillet, heat the oil on medium to relatively low heat.
3. Add minced garlic and grated ginger to the skillet and cook for 1 minute until fragrant.
4. Take the marinated tofu cubes and add them to the skillet. Cook until both sides are golden brown.
5. Take out and place aside the tofu from the skillet.
6. In the same skillet, add chopped vegetables and stir-fry until tender-crisp.
7. Return tofu to the skillet and toss with the vegetables until heated through.
8. Serve vegetable stir-fry over cooked brown rice or quinoa.

4. Quinoa Stuffed Bell Peppers

Ingredients:

- Four large bell peppers (remove the seed and cut into two).
- 1 cup cooked quinoa
- 1 can (15 ounces) black beans, drained and rinsed
- 1 cup diced tomatoes
- 1 cup corn kernels
- 1 teaspoon chili powder
- 1/2 teaspoon cumin
- Salt and pepper to taste
- Shredded cheese (optional)

Instructions:

1. Preheat the oven to 375°F (190°C).

2. In a large mixing bowl, combine cooked quinoa, black beans, diced tomatoes, corn kernels, chili powder, cumin, salt, and pepper.
3. Stuff each bell pepper half with the quinoa mixture.
4. Place stuffed bell peppers in a baking dish and cover with aluminum foil.
5. Bake in the preheated oven for 30-35 minutes, or until peppers are tender.
6. If using cheese, remove foil and sprinkle shredded cheese over the stuffed peppers during the last 5 minutes of baking.
7. Serve hot and enjoy this flavorful and nutritious meal.

5. Lentil Soup

Ingredients:

- 1 cup dried lentils
- 4 cups vegetable broth (low-sodium)
- 1 onion, diced
- 2 carrots, diced
- 2 stalks celery, diced
- 2 cloves garlic, minced
- 1 teaspoon dried thyme
- 1 teaspoon dried oregano
- Salt and pepper to taste
- Fresh lemon juice for serving

Instructions:

1. Rinse lentils under cold water and drain.
2. In a large pot, combine lentils, vegetable broth, diced onion, diced carrots, diced celery, minced garlic, dried thyme, and dried oregano.

3. Bring the mixture to a boil, then reduce heat and simmer for 25-30 minutes, or until lentils and vegetables are tender.

4. Season with salt and pepper to taste.

5. Serve hot with a squeeze of fresh lemon juice for added flavor.

6. Zucchini Noodles with Marinara Sauce

Ingredients:

- 4 medium zucchinis
- 2 cups marinara sauce (low-acid or homemade)
- 2 tablespoons olive oil
- 2 cloves garlic, minced
- 1 teaspoon dried oregano
- Salt and pepper to taste

- Grated Parmesan cheese for serving (optional)

Instructions:

1. Using a spiralizer or vegetable peeler, create noodles from the zucchinis.
2. In a big pan or skillet, heat the oil on medium to relatively low heat.
3. Add minced garlic and dried oregano to the skillet and cook for 1 minute until fragrant.
4. Add zucchini noodles to the skillet and sauté for 2-3 minutes until tender-crisp.
5. Pour marinara sauce over the zucchini noodles and toss to coat evenly.
6. Cook for an additional 2-3 minutes until heated through.
7. Season with salt and pepper to taste.

8. Serve hot with grated Parmesan cheese if desired.

7. Spinach and Ricotta Stuffed Shells (as listed above without meat)

8. Veggie Fried Rice

Ingredients:

- 2 cups cooked brown rice, cooled
- 2 tablespoons sesame oil
- 2 cloves garlic, minced
- 1 cup mixed vegetables (such as peas, carrots, and bell peppers)
- 2 green onions, chopped
- 2 tablespoons low-sodium soy sauce
- 1 teaspoon grated ginger
- 2 eggs, lightly beaten (optional)

Instructions:

1. In a big pan or skillet, heat the oil on medium to relatively low heat.
2. Add minced garlic to the skillet and cook for 1 minute until fragrant.
3. Add mixed vegetables to the skillet and stir-fry until tender-crisp.
4. Push vegetables to one side of the skillet and add beaten eggs to the other side (if using). Scramble until cooked through, then mix with the vegetables.
5. Add cooked brown rice to the skillet and toss to combine with the vegetables and eggs.
6. Stir in low-sodium soy sauce and grated ginger, mixing well.
7. Stir consistently, cook for two or three minutes.

8. Garnish with chopped green onions before serving.

9. Chickpea and Vegetable Curry

Ingredients:

- 1 tablespoon olive oil
- 1 onion, diced
- 2 cloves garlic, minced
- 1 tablespoon grated ginger
- 2 tablespoons curry powder
- 1 can of chickpeas, washed and sieved
- 1 can (14 ounces) diced tomatoes
- 1 can (14 ounces) coconut milk
- Assorted vegetables (such as cauliflower, spinach, and bell peppers), chopped
- Cooked brown rice for serving

Instructions:

1. In a big pan or skillet, heat the oil on medium to relatively low heat.
2. Add diced onion, minced garlic, and grated ginger to the pot. Sauté until onion is translucent.
3. Add the curry powder and stir until the aroma comes out, do that for about one minutes.
4. Stir in the diced tomatoes, coconut milk and chickpeas. Stir to combine.
5. Add assorted vegetables to the pot and simmer for 15-20 minutes, or until vegetables are tender.
6. Season with salt and pepper to taste.
7. Serve chickpea and vegetable curry over cooked brown rice.

10. Spinach and Mushroom Pasta

Ingredients:

- 8 ounces whole wheat spaghetti
- 2 tablespoons olive oil
- 2 cloves garlic, minced
- 8 ounces mushrooms, sliced
- 4 cups fresh spinach leaves
- 1/4 cup grated Parmesan cheese
- Salt and pepper to taste

Instructions:

1. Cook the whole wheat spaghetti according to the package instructions. Drain and set aside.
2. In a big pan or skillet, heat the oil on medium to relatively low heat.
3. Add minced garlic to the skillet and cook for 1 minute until fragrant.

4. Add sliced mushrooms to the skillet and cook until browned and tender.

5. Add the fresh spinach leaves and heat until they wilt.

6. Add cooked spaghetti to the skillet and toss to combine with the vegetables.

7. Season with salt and pepper to taste.

8. Serve hot, garnished with grated Parmesan cheese.

11. Baked Chicken Parmesan (with low-acid marinara sauce)

Ingredients:

- 4 boneless, skinless chicken breasts
- 1 cup whole wheat breadcrumbs
- 1/2 cup grated Parmesan cheese
- 1 teaspoon dried Italian seasoning

- Salt and pepper to taste
- 2 eggs, beaten
- 1 cup low-acid marinara sauce
- 1/2 cup shredded mozzarella cheese

Instructions:

1. Preheat the oven to 375°F (190°C). Lightly grease a baking dish.
2. In a shallow bowl, combine whole wheat breadcrumbs, grated Parmesan cheese, dried Italian seasoning, salt, and pepper.
3. Coat each chicken breast with the breadcrumb mixture after dipping it into the b eaten eggs.
4. Place breaded chicken breasts in the prepared baking dish.

5. Bake in the preheated oven for 25-30 minutes, or until chicken is cooked through and golden brown.

6. Remove from the oven and spoon low-acid marinara sauce over each chicken breast.

7. Sprinkle shredded mozzarella cheese over the sauce.

8. Return to the oven and bake for an additional 5-10 minutes, or until cheese is melted and bubbly.

9. Serve hot, garnished with chopped fresh basil if desired.

12. Vegetable and Tofu Stir-Fry

Ingredients:

- 14 ounces firm tofu, drained and cubed
- 2 tablespoons soy sauce (low-sodium)

- 1 tablespoon cornstarch

- 2 tablespoons olive oil

- 2 cloves garlic, minced

- 1 teaspoon grated ginger

- Assorted vegetables (such as broccoli, bell peppers, and snap peas), chopped

- Cooked brown rice or quinoa for serving

Instructions:

1. In a small bowl, toss tofu cubes with soy sauce and cornstarch until evenly coated.
2. In a big pan or skillet, heat the oil on medium to relatively low heat.
3. Add minced garlic and grated ginger to the skillet and cook for 1 minute until fragrant.
4. When the tofu cubes are marinated, add them to the skillet and fry them until golden all over.

5. Take out the tofu and place it aside in a skillet.

6. In the same skillet, add chopped vegetables and stir-fry until tender-crisp.

7. Return tofu to the skillet and toss with the vegetables until heated through.

8. Serve vegetable and tofu stir-fry over cooked brown rice or quinoa.

13. Eggplant and Zucchini Lasagna

Ingredients:

- 1 large eggplant, sliced lengthwise
- 2 medium zucchinis, sliced lengthwise
- 2 cups low-acid marinara sauce
- 2 cups low-fat ricotta cheese
- 1/4 cup grated Parmesan cheese
- 1 egg

- 1 teaspoon dried Italian seasoning
- Salt and pepper to taste
- 1 cup shredded mozzarella cheese

Instructions:

1. Preheat the oven to 375°F (190°C). Lightly grease a baking dish.
2. Lay eggplant and zucchini slices on a baking sheet lined with parchment paper. Sprinkle with salt and let sit for 10-15 minutes to release excess moisture.
3. Pat dry the eggplant and zucchini slices with paper towels.
4. In a mixing bowl, combine low-fat ricotta cheese, grated Parmesan cheese, egg, dried Italian seasoning, salt, and pepper.

5. Spread a thin layer of low-acid marinara sauce on the bottom of the prepared baking dish.

6. Layer eggplant and zucchini slices on top of the sauce.

7. Spread half of the ricotta mixture over the vegetable layer.

8. Repeat layers with remaining marinara sauce, eggplant, zucchini, and ricotta mixture.

9. Top with shredded mozzarella cheese.

10. Put the baking dish in the oven for thirty minutes in a preheated oven with the foil covering it.

11. Remove foil and bake for an additional 15-20 minutes, or until cheese is melted and bubbly.

12. Before serving, allow the lasagna to cool for a few minutes.

14. Baked Portobello Mushrooms with Quinoa
Salad

Ingredients:

- 4 large portobello mushrooms, stems removed
- 2 tablespoons balsamic vinegar
- 2 tablespoons olive oil
- 2 cloves garlic, minced
- Salt and pepper to taste
- 2 cups cooked quinoa
- 1 cup cherry tomatoes, halved
- 1/4 cup chopped fresh basil
- 1/4 cup crumbled feta cheese (optional)

Instructions:

1. Preheat the oven to 375°F (190°C). Lightly grease a baking sheet.

2. Combine the balsamic vinegar, olive oil, minced garlic, salt, and pepper in a small bowl.

3. Place portobello mushrooms on the prepared baking sheet.

4. Brush both sides of the mushrooms with the balsamic vinegar mixture.

5. Bake in the preheated oven for 15-20 minutes, or until mushrooms are tender.

6. In a mixing bowl, combine cooked quinoa, halved cherry tomatoes, chopped fresh basil, and crumbled feta cheese (if using).

7. Spoon quinoa salad into the baked portobello mushrooms.

8. Serve hot and enjoy this flavorful and nutritious dinner option.

ACID REFLUX SMOOTHIES

1. Banana Ginger Smoothie

Ingredients:

- 1 ripe banana
- 1/2 cup Greek yogurt (low-fat or dairy-free)
- 1 teaspoon grated ginger
- 1 tablespoon honey (optional)
- 1/2 cup almond milk (or any non-citrus non-dairy milk)
- Handful of ice cubes

Instructions:

1. Peel and slice the ripe banana.

2. In a blender, combine banana slices, Greek yogurt, grated ginger, honey (if using), almond milk, and ice cubes.

3. Blend until smooth and creamy.

4. Pour into a glass and enjoy

2. Papaya Pineapple Smoothie

Ingredients:

- 1 cup ripe papaya, diced
- 1/2 cup pineapple chunks
- 1/2 cup coconut water
- Juice of 1/2 lime
- Handful of ice cubes

Instructions:

1. In a blender, combine diced papaya, pineapple chunks, coconut water, lime juice, and ice cubes.
2. Blend until smooth and creamy.
3. Pour into a glass and enjoy

3. Berry Spinach Smoothie

Ingredients:

- 1/2 cup mixed berries
- 1 cup fresh spinach leaves
- 1/2 cup Greek yogurt (low-fat or dairy-free)
- 1 tablespoon chia seeds
- 1/2 cup almond milk (or any non-citrus non-dairy milk)
- Handful of ice cubes

Instructions:

1. In a blender, combine mixed berries, fresh spinach leaves, Greek yogurt, chia seeds, almond milk, and ice cubes.
2. Blend until smooth and creamy.
3. Pour into a glass and enjoy

4. Banana Oatmeal Smoothie

Ingredients:

- 1 ripe banana
- 1/4 cup rolled oats
- 1 tablespoon almond butter
- 1/2 teaspoon ground cinnamon
- 1/2 cup Greek yogurt (low-fat or dairy-free)
- 1/2 cup almond milk (or any non-citrus non-dairy milk)
- Handful of ice cubes

Instructions:

1. Peel and slice the ripe banana.
2. In a blender, combine banana slices, rolled oats, almond butter, ground cinnamon, Greek yogurt, almond milk, and ice cubes.
3. Blend until smooth and creamy.
4. Pour into a glass and enjoy this filling and satisfying smoothie.

5. Coconut Mango Smoothie

Ingredients:

- 1 cup ripe mango, diced
- 1/2 cup coconut milk (canned, unsweetened)
- 1/2 cup Greek yogurt (low-fat or dairy-free)
- 1 tablespoon honey (optional)
- Handful of ice cubes

Instructions:

1. In a blender, combine diced mango, coconut milk, Greek yogurt, honey (if using), and ice cubes.
2. Blend until smooth and creamy.
3. Pour into a glass and enjoy.

6. Apple Cinnamon Smoothie

Ingredients:

- 1 apple, cored and diced
- 1/2 teaspoon ground cinnamon
- 1/4 teaspoon ground nutmeg
- 1/2 cup Greek yogurt (low-fat or dairy-free)
- 1/2 cup almond milk (or any non-citrus non-dairy milk)
- Handful of ice cubes

Instructions:

1. In a blender, combine diced apple, ground cinnamon, ground nutmeg, Greek yogurt, almond milk, and ice cubes.
2. Blend until smooth and creamy.
3. Pour into a glass and enjoy

7. Green Tea Smoothie

Ingredients:

- 1 cup brewed green tea, cooled
- 1/2 cup mixed berries
- 1/2 banana
- 1 tablespoon honey (optional)
- Handful of spinach leaves
- Handful of ice cubes

Instructions:

1. In a blender, combine brewed green tea, mixed berries, banana, honey (if using), spinach leaves, and ice cubes.
2. Blend until smooth and creamy.
3. Pour into a glass and drink.

8. Creamy Avocado Smoothie

Ingredients:

- 1/2 ripe avocado, peeled and pitted
- 1/2 cup Greek yogurt (low-fat or dairy-free)
- Juice of 1/2 lime
- 1 tablespoon honey (optional)
- 1/2 cup coconut water
- Handful of ice cubes

Instructions:

1. In a blender, combine ripe avocado, Greek yogurt, lime juice, honey (if using), coconut water, and ice cubes.
2. Blend until smooth and creamy.
3. Pour into a glass and enjoy.

9. Peach Ginger Smoothie

Ingredients:

- 1 cup ripe peaches, diced
- 1 teaspoon grated ginger
- 1/2 cup Greek yogurt (low-fat or dairy-free)
- 1 tablespoon honey (optional)
- 1/2 cup almond milk (or any non-citrus non-dairy milk)
- Handful of ice cubes

Instructions:

1. In a blender, combine diced peaches, grated ginger, Greek yogurt, honey (if using), almond milk, and ice cubes.
2. Blend until smooth and creamy.
3. Pour into a glass and enjoy.

10. Pineapple Mint Smoothie

Ingredients:

- 1 cup pineapple chunks
- 1/4 cup fresh mint leaves
- 1/2 cup coconut water
- Juice of 1/2 lime
- Handful of spinach leaves
- Handful of ice cubes

Instructions:

1. In a blender, combine pineapple chunks, fresh mint leaves, coconut water, lime juice, spinach leaves, and ice cubes.
2. Blend until smooth and creamy.
3. Pour into a glass and enjoy.

11. Blueberry Almond Smoothie

Ingredients:

- 1/2 cup blueberries (fresh or frozen)
- 1 tablespoon almond butter
- 1/2 cup Greek yogurt (low-fat or dairy-free)
- 1 tablespoon honey (optional)
- 1/2 cup almond milk (or any non-citrus non-dairy milk)
- Handful of spinach leaves

- Handful of ice cubes

Instructions:

1. In a blender, combine blueberries, almond butter, Greek yogurt, honey (if using), almond milk, spinach leaves, and ice cubes.
2. Blend until smooth and creamy.
3. Pour into a glass and enjoy.

12. Raspberry Lemon Smoothie

Ingredients:

- 1/2 cup raspberries (fresh or frozen)
- Juice of 1/2 lemon
- 1/2 cup Greek yogurt (low-fat or dairy-free)
- 1 tablespoon honey (optional)

- 1/2 cup almond milk (or any non-citrus non-dairy milk)
- Handful of spinach leaves
- Handful of ice cubes

Instructions:

1. In a blender, combine raspberries, lemon juice, Greek yogurt, honey (if using), almond milk, spinach leaves, and ice cubes.
2. Blend until smooth and creamy.
3. Pour into a glass and enjoy.

13. Kiwi Banana Smoothie

Ingredients:

- 2 kiwis, peeled and sliced
- 1 ripe banana

- 1/2 cup Greek yogurt (low-fat or dairy-free)
- 1 tablespoon honey (optional)
- 1/2 cup almond milk (or any non-citrus non-dairy milk)
- Handful of spinach leaves
- Handful of ice cubes

Instructions:

1. In a blender, combine sliced kiwis, ripe banana, Greek yogurt, honey (if using), almond milk, spinach leaves, and ice cubes.
2. Blend until smooth and creamy.
3. Pour into a glass and enjoy

14. Cherry Vanilla Smoothie

Ingredients:

- 1/2 cup cherries (fresh or frozen)
- 1/2 teaspoon vanilla extract
- 1/2 cup Greek yogurt (low-fat or dairy-free)
- 1 tablespoon honey (optional)
- 1/2 cup almond milk (or any non-citrus non-dairy milk)
- Handful of spinach leaves
- Handful of ice cubes

Instructions:

1. In a blender, combine cherries, vanilla extract, Greek yogurt, honey (if using), almond milk, spinach leaves, and ice cubes.
2. Blend until smooth and creamy.
3. Pour into a glass and enjoy.

15. Mango Banana Smoothie

Ingredients:

- 1 cup ripe mango, diced
- 1 ripe banana
- 1/2 cup Greek yogurt (low-fat or dairy-free)
- 1 tablespoon honey (optional)
- 1/2 cup coconut water
- Handful of ice cubes

Instructions:

1. In a blender, combine diced mango, ripe banana, Greek yogurt, honey (if using), coconut water, and ice cubes.
2. Blend until smooth and creamy.
3. Pour into a glass and enjoy

16. Peach Raspberry Smoothie

Ingredients:

- 1 cup ripe peaches, diced
- 1/2 cup raspberries (fresh or frozen)
- 1/2 cup Greek yogurt (low-fat or dairy-free)
- 1 tablespoon honey (optional)
- 1/2 cup almond milk (or any non-citrus non-dairy milk)
- Handful of spinach leaves
- Handful of ice cubes

Instructions:

1. In a blender, combine diced peaches, raspberries, Greek yogurt, honey (if using), almond milk, spinach leaves, and ice cubes.
2. Blend until smooth and creamy.
3. Pour into a glass and enjoy.

17. Watermelon Mint Smoothie

Ingredients:

- 1 cup watermelon chunks
- 1/4 cup fresh mint leaves
- Juice of 1/2 lime
- 1/2 cup coconut water
- Handful of spinach leaves
- Handful of ice cubes

Instructions:

1. In a blender, combine watermelon chunks, fresh mint leaves, lime juice, coconut water, spinach leaves, and ice cubes.
2. Blend until smooth and creamy.
3. Pour into a glass and enjoy.

18. Blueberry Kale Smoothie

Ingredients:

- 1/2 cup blueberries (fresh or frozen)
- 1/2 cup kale leaves, stems removed
- 1/2 cup Greek yogurt (low-fat or dairy-free)
- 1 tablespoon honey (optional)
- 1/2 cup almond milk (or any non-citrus non-dairy milk)
- Handful of ice cubes

Instructions:

1. In a blender, combine blueberries, kale leaves, Greek yogurt, honey (if using), almond milk, and ice cubes.
2. Blend until smooth and creamy.
3. Pour into a glass and enjoy .

19. Strawberry Banana Smoothie

Ingredients:

- 1/2 cup strawberries (fresh or frozen)
- 1 ripe banana
- 1/2 cup Greek yogurt (low-fat or dairy-free)
- 1 tablespoon honey (optional)
- 1/2 cup almond milk (or any non-citrus non-dairy milk)
- Handful of spinach leaves
- Handful of ice cubes

Instructions:

1. In a blender, combine strawberries, ripe banana, Greek yogurt, honey (if using), almond milk, spinach leaves, and ice cubes.
2. Blend until smooth and creamy.

3. Pour into a glass and enjoy this classic and nutritious smoothie.

20. Mixed Berry Smoothie

Ingredients:

- 1/2 cup mixed berries
- 1/2 cup Greek yogurt (low-fat or dairy-free)
- 1 tablespoon chia seeds
- 1 tablespoon honey (optional)
- 1/2 cup almond milk (or any non-citrus non-dairy milk)
- Handful of spinach leaves
- Handful of ice cubes

Instructions:

1. In a blender, combine mixed berries, Greek yogurt, chia seeds, honey (if using), almond milk, spinach leaves, and ice cubes.

2. Blend until smooth and creamy.

3. Pour into a glass and enjoy this antioxidant-rich and fiber-packed smoothie.

14-DAY MEAL PLAN

Day 1:

Breakfast: Banana Ginger Smoothie
Lunch: Quinoa Salad with Grilled Chicken
Dinner: Baked Salmon with Lemon and Herbs, Steamed Vegetables
Snack: Greek Yogurt with Honey

Day 2:

Breakfast: Berry Spinach Smoothie
Lunch: Veggie Fried Rice
Dinner: Lentil Soup, Whole Wheat Bread
Snack: Sliced Apple with Almond Butter

Day 3:

Breakfast: Papaya Pineapple Smoothie
Lunch: Spinach and Ricotta Stuffed Shells (meatless)

Dinner: Vegetable Stir-Fry with Tofu, Brown Rice
Snack: Carrot Sticks with Hummus

Day 4:

Breakfast: Banana Oatmeal Smoothie
Lunch: Lentil and Vegetable Curry
Dinner: Grilled Chicken Breast with Roasted
Vegetables
Snack: Greek Yogurt with Mixed Berries

Day 5:

Breakfast: Coconut Mango Smoothie
Lunch: Chickpea and Vegetable Curry
Dinner: Quinoa Stuffed Bell Peppers (meatless)
Snack: Whole Grain Crackers with Avocado

Day 6:

Breakfast: Apple Cinnamon Smoothie
Lunch: Vegetable and Tofu Stir-Fry, Brown Rice

Dinner: Eggplant and Zucchini Lasagna (meatless)
Snack: Sliced Peaches

Day 7:

Breakfast: Green Tea Smoothie
Lunch: Creamy Avocado Smoothie
Dinner: Chickpea and Vegetable Stir-Fry, Quinoa
Snack: Greek Yogurt with Granola

Day 8:

Breakfast: Peach Raspberry Smoothie
Lunch: Spinach and Tomato Linguine (meatless)
Dinner: Baked Chicken Parmesan with Low-Acid
Marinara Sauce, Steamed Broccoli
Snack: Celery Sticks with Peanut Butter

Day 9:

Breakfast: Mango Banana Smoothie
Lunch: Quinoa Salad with Black Beans and Corn

Dinner: Veggie Fried Rice with Tofu
Snack: Cottage Cheese with Pineapple

Day 10:

Breakfast: Blueberry Kale Smoothie
Lunch: Lentil Soup, Whole Wheat Bread
Dinner: Grilled Salmon with Quinoa Salad
Snack: Sliced Cucumber with Hummus

Day 11:

Breakfast: Strawberry Banana Smoothie
Lunch: Egg Salad Lettuce Wraps
Dinner: Zucchini Noodles with Marinara Sauce
(meatless)
Snack: Mixed Nuts

Day 12:

Breakfast: Cherry Vanilla Smoothie
Lunch: Caprese Salad with Whole Wheat Pita

Dinner: Chickpea and Vegetable Curry, Brown Rice

Snack: Sliced Bell Peppers with Guacamole

Day 13:

Breakfast: Watermelon Mint Smoothie

Lunch: Greek Salad with Grilled Chicken

Dinner: Spinach and Mushroom Pasta (meatless)

Snack: Greek Yogurt with Strawberries

Day 14:

Breakfast: Mixed Berry Smoothie

Lunch: Quinoa Stuffed Bell Peppers (meatless)

Dinner: Baked Portobello Mushrooms with Quinoa Salad

Snack: Banana with Almond Butter